STOP GETTING SICK

A Step-by-Step Guide to Drastically Reducing the Number of Colds You Get Each Year

By Brian Stamile

Table of Contents

To my Mom,
for teaching me that
knowledge is power.

*"There is one consolation in being sick.
And that is the possibility that you may recover
to a better state than you were ever in before."*
-Henry David Thoreau

Preface

Are you sick of being sick? Tired of the tissues, medications, and doctors' visits? Do you avoid sick people like the plague, even at the risk of offending them? Have you finally said to yourself, "Enough is enough!" but don't know what to do next? If you answered yes, then you've picked up the right book.

It can be miserable slogging through life dealing with chronic recurring colds. It effects your relationships, your work, your happiness and even your mental stability. I've been there, and it's awful. But luckily there is a solution, and despite what I'm sure is your initial skepticism (I would be skeptical too), IT ACTUALLY WORKS!

But there is a catch (there's always a catch), you must follow the instructions as closely as you possibly can. Think of this book as not just a set of instructions, think of it as a weapon --a weapon that will allow you to conquer your colds and take back your life -- for good!

A Silent Scourge

There is an epidemic in this country that no one is talking about. Millions of Americans are subject to it each and every day, we're all affected by it at one time or another, and no one is spared. I'm talking about colds. Each day, 2.5 million Americans become infected with a cold. In fact, the average American get 2-4 colds per year, which adds up to 913 million colds per year (most of which last for 4-5 days). But that's just an average. There are some whose colds last much longer before all their symptoms clear up. Some people get 12 or more colds per year. I used to be in this unlucky group, the most stricken of all, but I'll tell you my story later, along with of course how to break free from this cycle and loosen its control over your life.

An increasing number of Americans are getting what I refer to as chronic recurring colds. Now, why is this happening you may ask? Why is this number increasing? Why are we even getting these sicknesses in the first place? Why hasn't medical science cured this? It costs our economy billions each year in productivity and causes individuals billions of hours of misery in aggregate. Who dropped the ball here? We can put a man on the moon but we can't stop the sniffles?

The startling fact is that we (and by we I mean everyone - scientists, public health officials and the average person) have absolutely no idea. I'm not going to sit here and tell you I can somehow answer this question with certainty. As far as I can tell, the cause of this epidemic is completely unknown to anyone on the planet. Sure, there are some theories, but nothing has been proven.

Here are couple of theories. Throughout history, science has proven itself inept in this area of medicine, resulting in colds not being at the forefront in the minds of research scientists. It's difficult to get funding to research something that has been studied for centuries (perhaps millennia) where the only useful advice to result is wash your hands. The advice on cold prevention has been essentially unchanged since the dark ages, when cleaning yourself started to be connected to disease prevention.

For humanity, colds have simply become a fact of life, and since most people only get them a few times a year it isn't not a major area of concern for most people, after all, does each of us really care about the billions of wasted economic productivity? Of course not, but we do care about ourselves and feeling optimal, and not losing days to sickness,

But I'm guessing since you bought this book that you're not one of these people who only get sick a couple of times a year. You're more likely to fall into the poor unfortunate category of people that suffer from colds often (more often than two or three times a year). You'd be ecstatic just to reduce the length of your colds to a few days. Sure, you've heard of people getting over colds and feeling better within 24 hours, but that's not the case for everyone. I'm here to tell you, I know your pain and I can help! Simply read on with an open mind.

Is This Book for Me?

If you are getting a significant number of colds each year (and by significant, I mean more than two per year) then this book can help you. Be aware, the purpose of this system is not to reduce the duration of colds. Typically, when this system is followed properly, cold duration decreases by a day or two, but the main goal of this book is to prevent colds from happening in the first place. There may be times when you get a cold and it lasts just as long as before you began the system. If you are someone that can do the same quick task each morning and night to help prevent colds then this book is for you. It may sound a bit daunting to do a task twice a day every day, but I think you'll find it will take very little discipline or will power because once you see how effective the system is, you will want to continue. The only caveat to this is that once the system has been effective for a long period of time, you may feel you are over that dark time of your life and you can stop the system entirely. This sadly is not the case, you must continue with this system forever in order to prevent colds. Think of this as a long-term investment in good health.

What Do You Know?

So you may be asking yourself, why should I believe him? Am I a doctor with advanced research? Absolutely NOT! However, you should believe me because I have been where you are now, I have come through the other side, and now I only get 1-2 colds a year.

Just How Effective Is This System?

The system described in this book WILL significantly lower the number of colds you get each and every year. Keep in mind that it will not prevent you from ever getting another cold again.

If you only get one cold a year, it may prevent that cold from occurring but that is unlikely. This system is meant to simply reduce the amount of colds you get each year.

My Story

My entire life I have always gotten colds more frequently than the average person, and often at the worst times (on vacation, during finals in college, etc.). It wasn't until I was 26 that for some reason I began getting colds once a month like clockwork, each and every month without exception.

The first symptom was always the same. I would start feeling inexplicably energetic for about a day, and then I would get drowsy for a few days and need to sleep much more than normal. Then, sure enough, my throat would start to tickle, gradually getting worse until it became extremely painful. Next, my nose would get stuffed up for about five days before becoming a hacking cough that would last for around 10 days. In total, the symptoms would last for anywhere between 2 and 3 weeks. Now, if this condition only lasted a few months I wouldn't have been very upset, but the fact was that it went on for YEARS and nearly destroyed my life in the process.

In truth, I rarely took sick days from work, because one sick day would simply not do it. I'd have to take weeks off at a time and I would not have been able to keep my job had I done that! I was miserable. It affected my relationships, and sometimes my desire to attend social events. It got to the point where if I knew someone was sick at an event, I would make up an excuse and leave, because I knew that I would likely catch that cold. None of this is an exaggeration. I even documented the dates I started feeling symptoms and when I felt better to record the frequency and duration. The startling thing was the clockwork-like nature of it all.

This went on for 3 years with no explanation and no cure. My work life was suffering, my home life was suffering, and I was at my wits end. During this time I tried everything to cure it. I read numerous books on cold prevention and all would site the same science and make the same recommendations. I talked to doctors, I talked to friends, I talked to people I had just met. Anything I could do to get a new tip or trick I hadn't tried before. I'll spare you the full list of things I tried because it's extremely extensive and I'm sure you already know or have tried many of them and know that they do not work. vitamin C, iron, even the stuff that logically seems to work is a total waste of time. Hand washing, although not a bad idea, didn't do the trick. Hand sanitizer, sleeping more, exercising a lot, eating tons of greens - many of these things are great for you, but none solved the underlying problem and were able to get me back even to anywhere near a normal cold frequency rate.

Even avoiding sick people didn't work as well as you might think. I tried them all with as much intensity as I possibly could, until two treatments when combined together finally worked. I stuck with it, and for the last 3 years, I have only gotten 1-2 colds per year (and the majority of those were right after air travel, which is a particularly high risk situation for colds).

What really convinced me that this wasn't just a coincidence was that it wasn't a gradual improvement. I went from colds once a month lasting for two and a half weeks to colds only once or twice a year as soon as I began following the system I describe in this book. Needless to say, I was ecstatic, I think about it every day how I was in such a dark place only to be reborn. It was almost a religious experience, and when I think about my current situation in life, it always occurs to me that I'm infinitely better off than during that dark multi-year period of constant sickness. I'm still not getting sick like that anymore and it makes me feel like I've conquered my own life.

Now you may say, I'm only one person so all this so-called "evidence" is just anecdotal and therefore may not work for me. My recommendation is that you gain a full understanding of the system before passing judgment, and try it for yourself before deciding that it doesn't work for you. You may be surprised!

Why is This System Better Than Other Cold Prevention Tips?

If I had to guess, it would be because other cold prevention tips attempt to address the underlying problem as something you are doing wrong, such as not enough sleep, stress, low Vitamin C, and so on. However, those who get sick often are usually living a very similar life to the rest of the population – except they're getting sick more!

It's true that I don't know exactly why this is happening to you, but I can say that this system is not focused on some internal microscopic effect like you might hear about in a doctor's office. Instead, it focuses on the physical removal of cold viruses and allergens before you're infected so that they don't have the opportunity to harm you.

The Importance of Commitment

As mentioned earlier, the most crucial part of the system is sticking with it. Give it 2-3 months before deciding it doesn't work, and follow the system carefully. It should take effect within 1-3 weeks of starting. A few days simply will not do. The key here is commitment. If you commit, you will succeed and your life will become much healthier.

A Brief Overview of the System

There are two parts to this system, both of which must be done in conjunction with one another to have the highest likelihood of success. First, I'll go over the most important part of the system and the only part that must be done daily. Then I will proceed in describing the second part. Please don't be discouraged by the amount of detail, as it is in your best interest so that you 100% understand exactly how to carry out this system in your day-to-day life.

Part 1: Keeping Your Nose Cold Free

The overwhelming majority of cold viruses enter through the nose, so the goal of Part 1 is to wash away any cold viruses or allergens that may have entered your nasal passageway twice a day. This prevents the virus from having enough time to attach to the lining of your sinuses and begin an infection.

STEP 1: PURCHASE EQUIPMENT AND SUPPLIES

I know, I know, you already bought this book and now you need to buy more stuff! First, let me reassure you that I have absolutely no connections with the companies that manufacture any of the items I'm suggesting that you purchase. I will also say that although this system does cost a small amount of money on a continual basis, it will pay for itself many times over in the form of reduced doctor visit costs, lower over the counter drug costs and reduced spending on cold remedies and therapies. Consider it an investment in you, and eventually it will be something you are happy to spend money since you will feel the benefits.

The other thing I'd like to stress is that it's crucial that you purchase the exact items I recommend. You may want to save a bit of money by buying similar substitutes or generic brands. DO NOT DO THIS as I cannot vouch for any products besides the ones I recommend in this book. This rule applies especially to the pre-mixed packets.

First, purchase two NeilMed Sinus rinse squeeze bottles and two Neilmed NasaDock Plus drying stand with Packet Storage from your local pharmacy or online. Also purchase at least 100 Neilmed Sinus Rinse pre-mixed packets. I always purchase these in batches of 250 to save money.

Despite the savings you may find online, I suggest buying these items from your pharmacy for the first time, so you can get started as soon as you possibly can.

Purchase at least three One Gallon plastic jugs of distilled water from your local supermarket or pharmacy. Make sure it's distilled water and not spring water. The distillation method or brand does not matter, the cheapest distilled water you can find is just fine. I buy at least five at a time and when I get down to two I purchase more so that I never run the risk of running out. The same thing goes for the pre-mixed packets. Once I get down to about 100 packets left, I purchase more.

To recap, you will need the following to begin this system:

- (2) NeilMed Sinus Rinse Squeeze Bottles
- (250) Neilmed Pre-mixed packets
- (2) Neiled NasaDock Plus Drying Stand
- (3) 1 Gallon Plastic Jugs of Distilled Water

STEP 2: SETTING UP YOUR EQUIPMENT

Store the gallons of distilled water in an area where they won't get dusty (inside a cupboard or drawer works great). If you don't have an adequate cupboard or drawer space, put each container inside a plastic grocery bag and tie the top so that dust can't get in. Next, put two of the one-gallon jugs in your refrigerator and let them cool for two hours before using them. Aim to always have two full gallons in your refrigerator if you have the refrigerator space.

Next, follow the Neilmed NasaDock drying stand setup instructions and place them on a counter or in a drawer or cupboard. DO NOT put them in your bathroom or kitchen. Now, open your squeeze bottles, give them a rinse with water in your sink, and you're ready to go. You'll notice in the instructions that come with the squeeze bottles that they recommend you use distilled or previously boiled water to clean them. I haven't figured out a way of actually doing this economically so I rinse them with tap water. However, if you can, I would encourage you to clean them in distilled or previously boiled water if possible, even bottled water would be better than tap. If you feel the need to clean the bottles with soap, be very careful to rinse them extremely thoroughly afterward (even the slightest amount of soap residue will burn if it goes through your nose and could be damaging). I recommend not cleaning these with soap for that reason.

STEP 3: READ THE FORMAL INSTRUCTIONS!

This step is VERY IMPORTANT. It's possibly the most important step. This book is similar to the actual instruction manual that comes with the squeeze bottles, but I still think it is crucial to read the formal instructions. Read them very carefully and thoroughly and follow them exactly. If not followed correctly, you could hurt yourself.

STEP 4: FREQUENCY

The key to this system working properly is consistency, and you must do this every day without exception no matter what. Use the squeeze bottle once after you wake up and once before going to sleep, no exceptions! Do not use it more than twice in one day, unless you have recently interacted with a sick person or were with a group of people where some were known to have colds. Also increase the frequency if you start feeling a cold coming on. If any of the above situations occurs, use the squeeze bottle as soon as you can after the interactions or immediately after you start feeling symptoms. Also avoid using it again within two hours of your last use to avoid discomfort from overuse. Three times per day is the ideal frequency if you are in a situation where someone sick is near you on a continual basis, such as a coworker at work. Three times is also appropriate if you start feeling cold symptoms coming on.

STEP 5: CLEANLINESS IS NEXT TO GODLINESS

Wash your hands thoroughly with soap and water. If using soap in the bottles, be sure to rinse thoroughly as residue may cause discomfort in your nasal passages.

STEP 6: FILL 'ER UP

Fill one squeeze bottle up with distilled water that has been chilled for at least 2 hours in your refrigerator. Open one of the pre-mixed packets and pour all of its contents into the squeeze bottle, being careful not to spill the salt mixture.

STEP 7: THINGS ARE HEATING UP

Microwave the filled bottle only (do not microwave the black nozzle that screws onto the squeeze bottle). Microwave time vary based on your specific appliance. I recommend setting your microwave to HIGH and starting with 40 seconds test the water temperature then add on 15 second increments until you identify the amount of time needed to make the liquid slightly above lukewarm temperature but NOT steaming hot. To test the temperature, put your thumb over the hole in the top of the bottle and turn it upside down so you can feel the liquid. If the water is still cold or feels hot, it is not the correct temperature. Either continue microwaving or wait for it to cool down. Remember slightly above lukewarm is perfect. And don't use it if the water feels hotter than that, it can hurt you!

STEP 8: SHAKE, SHAKE, SHAKE

Once you've tested the temperature and it feels only slightly warm, make a note of the number of seconds it took your microwave to get it to that exact temperature so that you remember for next time. With the black top still not screwed on, put your thumb over the hole hold the bottle firmly and shake it hard for at least 10 seconds. You're doing this to dissolve the salt evenly in the water and to make sure the warm water is an even temperature throughout the bottle.

STEP 9: THE BIG SQUEEZE

Screw the black nozzle back on the bottle and ensure that it is tight. This is important because sometimes these bottles allow extra air through the top, which will hurt the effectiveness of this step. At your bathroom sink, hold the bottle in your right hand and put it up to your right nostril. It shouldn't be pressed hard against your nostril, just the minimum amount of force needed to make a seal. Next, squeeze gradually with your thumb and middle finger on either side with your dominant hand, until the two meet, then stop to allow the water to flow through your nose and drain out the other nostril into the sink. You do not need to tilt your head, just hang forward slightly so that you are over the sink and the water can drain without making a mess. If you find this too difficult to perform comfortable keep at it, it gets easier over time.

The key here is to remember two things: 1. Test the temperature of the water. If it's too hot or too cold, stop Immediately and return to the fridge or microwave. DO NOT use the squeeze bottle until it's the appropriate temperature 2. Do not squeeze hard. Squeeze as softly as possible with your dominant hand while still causing the water to flow. Avoid the tendency to squeeze hard. If you notice that it's draining between a gap between your nose and the black nozzle, push the nozzle into your nose slightly more firmly. Once your thumb and middle finger have come together by squeezing the bottle, pull the bottle away from your nose and release your fingers. The bottle's water line should now be at about 50%.

STEP 10: BLOW IT OUT YOUR NOSE

The key here is to not cover or press one nostril before blowing out. I hesitate to use the word blow because it's really more like breathing out that I am asking you to do. DO NOT blow hard and DO NOT cover or press a nostril. Simply breath out gently with your mouth closed through both nostrils. Some weird stuff may come out, which is normal. Grab a tissue if you need to for easy clean up.

STEP 11: REPEAT WITH THE OTHER NOSTRIL

Repeat the same process with the left nostril, still using your dominant hand to squeeze with your middle finger and thumb. Do not feel like you need to use the entire contents of the bottle. If you keep squeezing and stopping and starting again, you may create spurts of pressure which may feel good but are not necessarily good for you. The key here is you want consistent pressure. Breathe out through your nose again gently without covering or closing a nostril, then use a tissue for cleanup.

STEP 12: AFTER THE SQUEEZE

Breath out through both nostrils slowly in a slow sustained fashion. You may also want to bend forward to allow any excess water to drain out. Using a couple tissues after to clean up is always a good idea.

STEP 13: RINSE THE BOTTLE

Rinse the bottle and the nozzle then shake out the bottle as much as you can before putting the bottle back on the stand upside down for draining. If using soap, I'd recommend against using dish soap such as Joy or Ajax. Something gentler, like Meyer's Hand Soap, would be better as it will leave less of a soapy residue. Again, be sure to rinse thoroughly if using soap.

STEP 14: WASH YOUR HANDS AGAIN TO COMPLETE PROCESS

Wash your hands again with soap and water. You're done!

Quick Recap

We just covered the steps involved in the first half of this cold prevention system. Essentially, it involves using the NeilMed Sinus Rinse squeeze bottle twice a day, every day, forever. Don't be discouraged by the word forever, you won't mind at all because this system works.

The key points to remember:

- Only use slightly warm water

- Squeeze gently

- Don't blow your nose hard

Additional Required Steps:

Cleaning the drying stands

Each month you should carefully clean the two drying stands in the sink with soap and water and a sponge or paper towel. Every 2-3 months replace the squeeze bottles entirely.

Restock your supplies

Buy more distilled water when needed. You'll go through this quickly so feel free to stock up if you have the space or if it is on sale. Be sure to purchase more pre-mixed packets before you're out (I re-order when I'm down to about 100 packets left just to be sure).

Tips and Tricks:

Don't share bottles with others! Even your husband or kids. Label them if you have to. They are your ticket to health, guard them well.

Restock in advance! Whether it's water, packets or tissues packets, make sure you don't run out. If you miss a day or two, you will lose momentum and very likely will not go back to the system. Stick with it, even if you're tired. It will be worth it.

Frequently Asked Questions

What's with the two setups of supplies?

It usually takes more than 12 hours for one squeeze bottle to completely dry out, even when hanging upside down (24 hours is best). It's important that you alternate the bottles, so essentially you'll always use the same bottle in the morning and the same bottle at night. I recommend using the one on the left in the morning and the one on the right at night, just so you remember more easily. Label them if you need to!

Should the solution be running down the back of my throat?

If water is trickling down the back of your throat during use, try breathing slowly in and out through your mouth during use. This will seem odd at first, but it will prevent the water from draining into the back of your throat.

What if it's burning my nose during use?

There are a few reasons why this might occur: (1) The water is either too hot too cold. (2) You are doing the process too frequently. (3) You didn't shake up the contents well enough. (4) You didn't use the entire packet. (5) You didn't fill the bottle to the line. (6) You used too much water or not enough. (7) There is soap residue remaining in the bottle.

What do I do if the solution won't go all the way through my nose?

Squeeze a little, then stop. Repeat until you're able to get it through, or stop and try again later. It's important not to increase your squeeze pressure.

What if my nose is leaking long after use?

Occasionally if you bend down later in the day, some water will pour out of your nose in a surprising way. This is normal. Just grab a tissue and clean up. You can prevent this from happening by doing a forward bend right after use for drainage.

What if acne develops around my nose?

If you happen to notice that you have a few more zits than usual around your nose, be sure to wash your face with soap immediately after performing the squeeze bottle process. I use the squeeze bottle before showering in the morning to kill two birds with one stone, but in the evening it's best to do it right before washing your face.

What if I don't have a microwave?

You can use a tea kettle to heat up the water, just be sure it's as clean as possible (rinse all soap out thoroughly before use). I'd also recommend doing some trial and error to figure out exactly how long it will take to heat up the exact amount of water you need, keep the stove on high, and time it with a stop watch or timer. To get the exact amount of water, fill the squeeze bottle to the line then pour the contents of the bottle into the kettle and place over heat. I'd also recommend using a thermometer at first to help you do this, as you don't want to pour very hot water into the squeeze bottle. Boiling water and plastic don't mix well! I'd recommend purchasing a cheap microwave if possible to avoid added time and waste.

How was this system created?

I tried dozens of cold prevention systems. I read books and articles on cold prevention, spoke with doctors and developed a lengthy list of dozens of potential solutions. Then for two years I tried them all as carefully as I could. I did each one to fruition to see if it would help, constantly documenting what, if any, the impact was of each. I approached each one with skepticism and did the best I could not to let my own desire to be cured cloud my judgement as to whether or not a particular system was effective. I left no stone unturned, even old wives tales, home remedies, everything from Native American remedies to following a variety of doctor's instructions. I even spoke with a psychologist about this to explore any possible psychosomatic causes. It was an extremely painstaking process, and ultimately these two methods were the only ones that had a noticeable impact.

Immediately after beginning this system, I stopped getting colds. I will still get either one or two colds a year, but these I attribute to being right after exposure to an extremely high-risk situation, such as taking lengthy vacation abroad or flying on an airplane. I also spent gobs of money on cold prevention systems, and this system is what I found worked, and boy did it.

Can't I just do this once a day?

No you cannot. Doing the process twice a day is crucial for success. I have tried doing it once a day and it does not have the desired effect. 24 hours is far too much time to accumulate allergens or viruses in your nose.

How long do I have to do this for?

Well, to be honest, the answer is forever. Don't let this prospect discourage you, once you see how well this works you really won't mind I'm sure of it.

What if there is a cold prevention system that works that I don't have to do every day?

Well, there may be, but I doubt it. This system works unbelievably well, and I believe once you try it and see its results, you will consider any other systems.

How can I maintain the discipline needed to do this process each and every day?

You must do this with a highly disciplined mindset. Try telling your significant other or roommate about what you're doing to hold you accountable, and so that they can remind you. Once you do it for a month it will become a habit and you'll do it without thinking.

Why do you think this works so well?

Again, I'm not a doctor, but I do have some theories. Most people contract colds through their nose. The virus enters on a microscopic droplet of mucus, is breathed in and attaches to the cells lining your nasal passageway. It sits there for a while and, after a day or so, the virus attacks and invades those cells and your body has an immune response, which result in all the symptoms you feel. The point here is that it takes a bit of time for it to invade the lining of your nose. This process works because it washes away the virus before it can attach and cause an immune response. This is also why it is important to do this frequently!

Another theory I have is that allergies and colds are more linked than most people are aware of, and you may initially have allergies due to something you breathed in, like dust mites pet dander or pollen. Your nose has a response to the allergen by creating more mucus to attempt to wash away the allergen. It also tries to protect the cells lining your nose from the allergen with a thick layer of mucus, but in doing so, it also causes a stuffed-up nose and too much mucus. This clogging up of your nose passageways causes old mucus to sit around for so long that it creates a perfect environment for a sinus infection to occur. Bacteria and viruses then grow in this clogged up stagnant environment, eventually resulting in an infection and your body responding to that infection with cold symptoms.

How long does this process take each day?

I have it down to science at this point, as I'm sure you will too eventually. At this point, I can do the whole process in about 2-3 minutes. Therefore it's really only a 4-6 minute commitment each day.

How soon before I should notice improvement?

Give it a few weeks. You will want to do the system long enough for you to notice that you are getting sick considerably less.

What do I do when traveling?

This is a tough one. Transporting the pre-mixed packets and squeeze bottle is easy enough, just be sure to keep them in a clean zip-lock bag to maintain cleanliness during travel. Make sure it's dry before putting it in the bag.

The distilled water is a little more difficult. You have a few options here. You can purchase distilled water at your destination, you can bring it with you (this is not advisable since distilled water is bulky and heavy). You can also purchase prefilled Neilmed sinus rinse squeeze bottles at many pharmacies, but this can be expensive and heavy for a one-time use, It may be worth it in a pinch and it beats getting sick! You can also use tap or bottled water and boil it then wait for it to cool off, then use as you would distilled water. This is a little tough because you have to find a way to boil the water in a clean sterile situation. The last option is my preferred option. I'll use bottled water purchased on location, keep the water bottle sealed, then put it in the sink of my hotel room with hot tap water running over it to heat up, after about 10 minutes the water in the bottle is usually warm enough to use. This situation is not ideal since you're not using distilled water, but it should work in a pinch.

Why distilled water?

There have been instances of people in certain areas of the United States using tap water in a neti pot and the water contained a bacteria that caused death when it got into their sinus cavity. To be safe, I suggest distilled water, and highly suggest not using tap water unless it is previously boiled. I can't stress this enough.

Do I have to keep the gallon of water in the fridge?

Yes, it will keep it pure and clean for longer. Remember you're opening this jug at least twice a day, and germs can enter the jug when it's open or seep through the seal when it's closed but not sealed. Keeping it in your fridge is a smart idea, as it also allows the water to stay at a consistent temperature so heating it up in your microwave or kettle will take exactly the same amount of time each time you do it.

Other Benefits to This System

Although this book may be entirely focused on cold prevention you may experience some additional benefits, such as allergy reduction, sleeping better, feeling less tired and more energetic, less frequent stuffed up nose, less frequent post nasal drip, fewer headaches, coughing less, less nasal sounding voice, less sneezing, increased alertness due to easier breathing and more oxygen inhalation and if you trim your nose hairs, it cleans them all away nicely. There are many more benefits that you may or may not experience!

Cost Calculation

When you add in the bottle replacements, pre-mixed packets use, tissues and distilled water use, the total is roughly $15 to $27 per month.

If the cost is worrying you, just remember this:

> *The greatest wealth is health.*
> *-Virgil*

Don't forget that getting colds is not free. Doctor visit costs add up, as do over-the-counter medications and cough drops. Commit to spending money on this for a few months and if it helps, you won't mind making room in your budget for this.

Part 2: Keeping Your Throat Cold Free

Cold viruses very often manifest in the throat, so the purpose of this section is to prevent viruses from infecting the throat by removing them thoroughly at the first sign of an invasion.

Overview of Part 2

I mentioned at the beginning of this book that using the NeilMed Sinus Rinse Squeeze bottles is only one part of the overall cold prevention system. Admittedly it's the most important and effective piece, however there is another part that I can't leave out and you definitely shouldn't either. Not unless you want to continue getting sick!

The main difference between Part 1 and Part 2 is that you don't have to do Part 2 every day. I only recommend you do every day, twice a day for the first two weeks of starting this whole journey. After the initial two weeks, you can begin doing this part of the system only if you feel a cold coming on. In summary, this part is based on your judgement and awareness of your own body to some extent.

What does it mean to start feeling sick? Well, it's a bit different for everyone. I explained earlier in the book how for me I became energetic, followed by tiredness, followed by throat pain. But for you it may be different. Here is a list of possible early signs you may see that indicate there is a cold lurking deep within. If you feel any of these at all, do this part of the system 3 times a day until symptoms subside.

1. Slight throat tingle
2. Throat pain when swallowing
3. Unexplained tiredness
4. Unexplained extra energy
5. Unexplained headache (if this is not common for you)
6. Sneezing fit
7. Coughing fit

8. Runny nose
9. Stuffy nose

In addition to the above, you should also do this if you feel you are extremely at risk of getting sick soon. What do I mean by this? Here are some examples that should trigger you to perform this part of the system for 3-4 days. These are also the situations that would warrant doing the Neilmed system 3 times a day for a short period of time:
1. Took a plane flight
2. Shared drinks with multiple people
3. Shared drinks with a known sick person
4. Kissed a sick person
5. Spent several hours in close proximity to a sick person

If any of the above situations occur, you should follow the system just as I describe below 3 times a day for 3 days straight for high-risk situations, or until symptoms subside.

Steps of Part 2

BUY SUPPLIES

Purchase a minimum of two bottles of 16.9 ounces of Colgate Peroxyl mouth wash. You also have the option of buying a generic mouthwash, but it must the label must say something along the lines of *compare to active ingredients in Peroxyl, CVS Pharmacy has a great store brand replacement that is significantly less expense. One bottle of 16.9 ounce Peroxyl costs between $8 and $13 dollars, and you need at least two. I recommend that you buy two so that as soon as you use one up you buy another, just like the distilled water and pre-mixed packets. DO NOT wait until you're almost out of Peroxyl to buy more, as timing is extremely important. You must use it as soon as you possibly can when you begin feeling a cold or have been in a high-risk situation, so you will not want to risk running out of Peroxyl when you begin feeling the start of cold symptoms. The earlier that you can use the Peroxyl when symptoms begin, the better, minutes really do matter.

USING THE PEROXYL

Take about a half ounce of Peroxyl (one swig) into your mouth (best to be in front of your sink). Tilt your head way back and gargle as deep in your throat and as forcefully as you can. Ensure that the Peroxyl is interacting with your tonsils and as far back in your throat as you can get it, but don't choke! Continue gargling for about 30-60 seconds or so (the longer the better) then swish around your mouth and teeth, then spit it out into the sink.

REPEAT THIS PROCESS

Do this once more. Gargle for a minimum of 30 seconds, swish and then spit.

CONTINUE TO SPIT IF NECESSARY

You'll notice that after a few seconds it foams up again in your mouth so continue to spit into the sink as needed. Feel free to take a sip of water and swish it around your mouth before spitting again.

SUMMARY

Now you know the second part of the system. In summary, it is gargling two times with Peroxyl mouthwash three times a day (preferably when you wake up, once in the middle of the day and again before bed) when you feel a cold coming on, or if you were in a high-risk situation for catching a cold. It's important not to skip this step.

Frequently Asked Questions

Why does this work?

Just like with the Neilmed squeeze bottle, there's no way to know for sure why it works, but my guess would be that the antiseptic qualities of the hydrogen peroxide kills any cold viruses or bacteria that is sitting on your tonsils or throat.

How did you come up with this system if the squeeze bottle was shown to be effective?

It's true that after I tested the Neilmed squeeze bottle treatment I stopped getting sick, although I did notice though that periodically my throat would get a tickle and although it wouldn't progress into a full blown cold, my throat sometimes began hurting as if I was coming down with a cold (which eventually went away on its own). I continued testing systems that focused on the throat and eventually came across this method, tested it, and sure enough as soon as my throat felt slightly off I would do this system and it would clear it up within a day or two.

What do I do while traveling?

Bring a bottle of Peroxyl with you! It is a small sized bottle and can be stowed in your checked luggage. I wouldn't recommend relying on buying it after you arrive at your destination, as you may have trouble finding it. If you're not checking luggage, pour it into a small clean travel sized bottle. When traveling, I still recommend maintaining a high standard of cleanliness, such as washing your hands often and using hand sanitizer or wipes. Don't forget to bring tissues with you!

Can't I just gargle Hydrogen Peroxide?

No, as Peroxyl is different. Not to mention, the Peroxyl mouthwash is meant to be used in your mouth, where as hydrogen peroxide is not designed for this purpose.

If this works so well, why isn't it more well-known?

I predict that it will be soon as more and more people read this book and put this system into practice.

Conclusion

We have now covered from beginning to end the entire system in detail for how you can finally stop chronic recurring colds from tormenting you.

Part One of this system involved using a Neilmed Sinus Rinse Squeeze bottle as a preventative measure twice a day, every day. Part Two involves gargling with a benzoyl peroxide based mouthwash (called Peroxyl) as soon as you feel a cold coming on, or if you have been in a high-risk situation. The most important thing to remember about this system is to stick with it for the long term!

I hope that after reading this book, you will move past any skepticism or apprehension that you may have about the system. Don't be discouraged by how simple and straightforward it is. After all, you won't know for yourself if it works until you try. Get started today and STOP GETTING SICK!

Spread the Word

Thank you so much for reading this book. I have a small favor to ask of you, the reader.

If you enjoyed this book, I'd really appreciate if you left an honest review about it on Amazon. It will take only a minute of your time, and it will mean the world to me. Every single review counts!

Thanks for your support!

Kind regards,
Brian